# Quick Guide

## How to Lose Fat and Shape your Body

**Claus Lauter**

cl publishing

Cape Town, South Africa

First edition

Copyright © Claus Lauter 2010

ISBN: 978-0-620-45994-5

Published by cl publishing, 3 Leeuwkop Street, Suite
102, Cape Town, South Africa

Design and layout by Claus Lauter

"There is only one way to climb a mountain
- step by step." - Unknown

I dedicate this book, with great respect, to the late Mrs. Traute Zimmermann who thought me discipline, respect and flexibility.

# TABLE OF CONTENTS

1

# INTRODUCTION

This book is about losing body fat and weight. It is a proven concept and worked very well for the author as well as for others.

It is not a 300 page book that explains the whole human biochemistry and gives you hundreds of cooking recipes. It is not a book that shows you how to lose 25 pounds in 7 days.

There are more than 60 ebooks on diet and fat loss on the Internet. And some of them are really good, some of them are crap, but most of the time they have too much information to deal with.

This book will give you the very basic rules and guidelines to reach your target in losing body fat while maintaining or even building muscles. This book should be easy and quick to read and to understand.

This book is written for the average person that has an 8 hours job, family and other tasks to fulfill.

There are enough other books, that make losing fat and sticking to your diet an impossible mission because it will require more time or money than you can invest.

The book is not full of scientific studies or complicated rules. It will demonstrate in a simple and understandable language what you can do to lose weight and become healthier.

# INTRODUCTION

- This book will not give you the Top 100 weight loss tips.

- It will not tell you to count calories.

- And of course this book will not make Mr. or Mrs. Universe out of you.

- It will only show you a lifestyle that will help you to lose fat, get in shape and live a healthier and more fitness orientated life.

- The diet and workout routines are easy to follow.

- A typical workout is quick, not more than 30-40 minutes per day.

- You have one day a week were you can eat whatever you want, even unhealthy junk food.

***

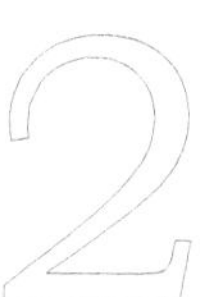

# SOME BACKGROUND INFORMATION

The human body is a very effective biological machine even though it's a very old machine and the basic program is still the same as it used to be in the stone-age.

Our ancestors were hunters and gatherers and did not have the chance to get their food in the supermarket at day and night times. Therefore they had to eat as much as possible whenever they had something. The body then stored the additional food as fat for times when food was not available.

And of course they tried to save energy whenever possible so they could survive the harsh environment.

Nowadays this old and nevertheless good idea still works and is the reason why two thirds of all US Americans are overweight. In industrialized countries, that excess body fat is unnecessary.

The best way to lose your body fat is: Eating! And... Fat doesn't make you fat, excess calories do.

So only eat the amount of food that you really need and not more than that. You also need to be active. With this setting you will able to beat the old, odd program in your brain.

You will eat 5-6 time a day, but only small portions and you will keep it easy. By doing this over a period of time your body will adapt to the new intake scheme.



This leads to the result of avoiding the yo-yo effect, you will see how to change your life style and your eating habits.

***

3

# SET YOUR GOAL

First of all you need to set a goal that you want to achieve. And it must be a goal that you really must approve of. It is not a figure on your scale but rather a picture in your mind. Stay realistic: You will not be Arnold Schwarzenegger or a super slim fitness model.

The easiest is to read some journals or newspaper or

browse the web and look out for people that have the shape that you are willing to have. Then cut this picture out and stick it into your wardrobe or next to your bathroom mirror.

Maybe even put a picture of your face on it. Make sure that you will see the picture every day. It needs to be burned into your brain.

If you can visualize this as a picture of you it is far easier to reach your target. And yes, it is a good idea to take a picture of your actual body and pin it next to your future body. It will later remind you where you started.

You mind and your will are your most important partners on the mission. Even more important than your diet, your supplements or your training plan.

You need to really believe in yourself and visualize the picture of your future shape. You are on a diffi-cult mission that will require a lot of discipline. And you need motivation. So be your own best buddy and build up your confidence to reach you goal.

But not only your picture is important. Also make sure that you know and understand the advantages of a healthier lifestyle. And there are many. I am sure you know at least some of them.

Here are some examples:

- reduced stress levels
- lower risk of heart disease
- lower risk of diabetes
- increased metabolic rate
- improved cholesterol levels
- lower risk of cardiovascular disease
- lower risk of high blood pressure
- lower risk of gallbladder disease
- improved digestion
- overall better feeling and well being
- more attractive to others
- more active
- boosted immune system
- more energy
- makes you stronger
- lower risk of injuries to your joints and chronic pain

- feeling better, both inside and outside
- more self-confidence and self-esteem
- you get involved with doing the things you love. e. g. sports, outdoor activities

You should set realistic goals. If you have gained weight and body fat over a couple of months or years, there is no way to lose it within a couple of days.

All diets telling you something like "Lose 14 pounds in 7 days" are absolute nonsense.

You will lose mainly water and then after a couple of days, your body will store the water again. All your effort was useless and you will tell yourself that this diet is not working for you.

Besides this: Up to 60% of the human body is water and it is not healthy to take too much water away as this will influence important functions in your body.

Perceive your goal as a medium to long term project It is important to set small goals along the way.

# SET YOUR GOAL

Don't say that you want to have 10% body fat when you are starting off with 32% plus.

Rather say: "I want to come down from obese to acceptable". For a woman that would be 26% for example. And then set a new goal of maybe 23% with which you have achieved a fitness level.

You will have more excitement, when you reach the next level and intermediate goal from time to time instead of waiting for the success of the final goal for a long time.

Do look on your scale and look in the mirror. We do not want to lose an exact amount of kilograms but rather shape the body.

And yes it will take some work, but the rewards are endless.

One thing that you must bear in mind: "Fat loss is simple, but it's not easy!"

If you do not have the motivation or the willpower,

then this program will not work for you. Have a positive and upbeat attitude.

I am convinced that you will be able to do it.

***

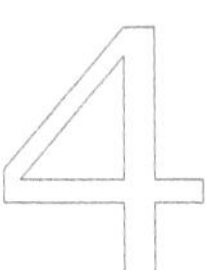

# LET`S GET STARTED

First of all we need a definition of fat. What does fat on your body mean? Every body needs fat. You cannot live without it, as fat has some important tasks to fulfill in your body.

But... you only need a bit of fat. And this is measured with a figure called Body Mass Index (BMI).

The body mass index is determined by your height and weight ratio.

It is your weight in pounds divided by your height in inches. If your BMI is higher than 30, you are considered obese, and should lose some fat.

The following table will give you an overview of body fat categories:

| Classification | Women (% fat) | Men (% fat) |
| --- | --- | --- |
| Essential Fat | 10-12% | 2-4% |
| Athletes | 14-20% | 6-13% |
| Fitness | 21-24% | 14-17% |
| Acceptable | 25-31% | 18-25% |
| Obese | 32% plus | 25% plus |

It will be a good idea to consult your doctor, if you are obese. A general check-up should be your starting point to get your blood pressure, cholesterol etc controlled.

Save and store the results for later. And if you doctor gives you the green light, it is time to start.

Set your start date and prepare for your first 12 weeks.

The first things are already done. You have a medical check-up and you have a realistic picture of your future body somewhere where you will see it. Speak to people about your plan and that you will reach your goal.

The more you do it the more you will be convinced to achieve it and of course others will expect to see your results in 3 months. So you are already on your mission.

***

5

# YOUR NEW FOOD HABITS

I do not know you, but you would not read this, if you food habits were perfect, because then you would not need this book.

So let's start with some easy and general hints on your new food habits:

# YOUR NEW FOOD HABITS

DO's and DON'T's

- Try to eat colorful.
  This means that the more colors the food on your plate has the better. Example: Sandwich: Salad (green), Tomato (red), full wheat toast (brown), low fat cheese (yellow), egg and low fat mayo (white)

- Your meals (lunch, dinner) should always include a source of protein and carbohydrates and some vegetables.

- The size of the carbohydrates and protein part should always be smaller than your fist. Example: portion of rice < size of your fist and chicken breast < size of your open palm

- Don't skip breakfast!

- You should always have some vegetables or salad with every lunch or dinner.

- You should eat at least 6 times as day, about every 3-4 hours. You need to eat, do not skip the meals. We want a constant blood sugar level over the day. This will prevent you from starving and having hunger attacks. So again, do not skip your meals and mid-morning or mid-afternoon snacks. You have to eat to lose fat!

- Try to prepare your food in advance, e.g. in the evening for the next day. Then your day will be more stress free. Always have some backup diet protein bars or fruit with you.

- You should drink lots of water: 2-3 liters a day. You will eat less and get rid of toxins in your body.

- Try to drink water in place of soft drinks and other flavored beverages.

- If you have a business lunch chose something from the menu that will fit your new habits. There are always some chicken and plain vegetables on the menu. Or just ask the waiter to ask the kitchen to prepare something for you.

YOUR NEW FOOD HABITS

- Do not drink any soft-drinks, fruit juices, full fat milk

- Avoid excess amounts of alcohol, like beer, wine, etc.

- Avoid food with added sugars

- Consider eating organic

- Don't buy processed or junk food

- You can drink as much (sugar-free) coffee or tea as you like.

- Do not add additional salt or sodium to your food.

- Do not eat carbohydrates in the evening after 7.00 pm. For late night craving make yourself a protein smoothie.

- Don't drink diet sports or energy drinks.

- Don't store unhealthy food in your home. You can't eat what you don't buy!

OK, this sounds bad, real bad. But it is not as bad as it seems because there is also good news for you.

Your diet will only be six days a week. On day seven you can eat what you want and as much as you want to eat. So once a week you will be given a real feast and you can enjoy all the food you love.

BUT... only once a week!!

You have to stick to this concept for at least 12 weeks. You body needed years to build up the fat that you carry around and is also used to the food intake you have given it. It will take your body a while to get used to the new scheme.

But believe me it is not too hard as the human body adjusts to the new situation quite quickly.

***

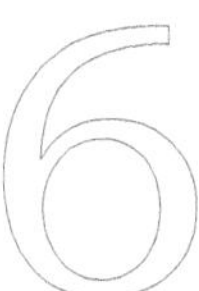

# GO SHOPPING

We will change your eating habits to a medium protein, medium carbohydrate and low fat lifestyle. So we need to go shopping for this.

Here are the basic shopping guidelines:

- Try to ban fat and hidden fat from you shop-ping cart.

- Only shop once a week and buy all food for the whole week. This will prevent you from being in the shop to often and making some wrong decisions.

- Take your shopping list with you and stick to it. Get what's on your list and get back home. This is not a recreational activity.

- Do not buy poor-quality junk foods.

- Buy fresh fruits and vegetables.

- Avoid processed meats like sausages.

- Do not hurry and do not go when everyone is rushed and busy. Rather go on a Sunday morning.

- Read the nutritional fact labels and notice how much fat and sodium is in the food.

- This is a fundamental rule of shopping: Do NOT shop when you are hungry. You only end up buying food like candy bars to feed your low sugar level.

- Do YOUR shopping. If you have to shop for your family and kids do it separately. Store your food separately. This is your food. This is your mission. It will be your success.

***

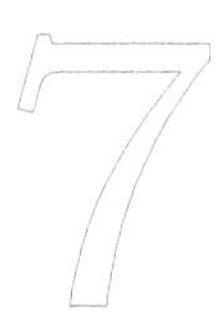

# THE SHOPPING LIST

(You do not need to buy everything at once.)

- Mineral water, Coffee, Tea
- Skinless chicken breasts
- Lean beef steak
- Turkey or Ostrich burgers
- Lean ground beef
- Old-fashioned oatmeal
- Bran Flakes

# THE SHOPPING LIST

- Whole-wheat bread
- Whole-wheat hamburger buns
- Whole-wheat spaghetti
- Whole-wheat flour
- Brown rice
- Salsa
- Soy sauce
- Lime juice
- Brown sugar
- Lemon juice
- Mixed nuts
- Ketchup
- Mustard
- Pepper
- Salt
- Paprika
- Garlic powder
- Cloves of fresh garlic
- Cumin
- Parsley
- Dill weed
- Celery
- Water chestnuts

- Dill pickles
- Spinach leaves
- Fresh tomatoes
- Cucumber
- Cauliflower
- Lettuce
- Onions
- Canned whole tomatoes
- Fresh mushrooms
- Canned kidney beans
- Basil
- Oregano
- Ginger
- Chili powder
- Extra virgin olive oil
- Balsamic vinaigrette
- Low-fat mayo
- Caesar dressing
- Cooking spray
- Blueberries
- Raspberries
- Apples
- Bananas

- Peaches
- Strawberries
- Pears
- Grapes
- Grated Parmesan cheese
- Low-fat cheese slices
- Fat-free sour cream
- Skim milk
- Low-fat cottage cheese
- Fresh eggs
- Egg substitute
- Low-fat yogurt
- Cream cheese
- Canned tuna in water
- Salmon fillet
- Trout
- Sugar-free syrup
- Fresh lime juice
- All-natural peanut butter
- Honey
- Peanuts
- Carrots
- Romaine lettuce

- Broccoli
- Sweet potatoes
- White potatoes

This food choice will give you a broad variety of possible meals.

There are lots of recipes on the web. But as we will keep it simple, you don't need to be a world famous chef.

***

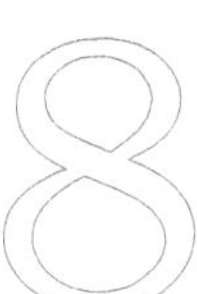

# A TYPICAL DAY OF THE DIET

6.00 am – 1 Glass of water, 1 Multivitamin, 2 Omega Oil tabs
(Uhh, what is this? Drugs? No! Stay tuned. I will explain the need for supplements later.)

8.00 am - breakfast after work out: 1 Glass of water, 1 sugar free coffee or tea, 1 small bowl of bran flakes, oats, muesli with fat free milk and hey, guess what: no sugar



10.00 am – mid-morning snack:  some fruit

        or a diet protein bar

        or a low carb whey protein shake


1.00 pm – lunch: 1 Glass of water, sandwich with brown toast, chicken breast, tomato, crisp salad, low fat cheese and low fat mayo


4.00 pm –   afternoon snack: handful of peanuts

        or a diet protein bar

        or a low carb whey protein shake


7.00 pm dinner - Grilled steak, steamed Broccoli, 3 cooked potatoes, Fat-free sour cream, Glass of water


9.00 pm – low-fat yogurt with banana and honey


You can vary with this as you want. But again, keep the portions small and eat at least 6 times a day. Stick to this Monday to Saturday.

And on Sundays take your family and friends out to a restaurant and enjoy your Lasagna, ice cream, chocolate, muffins etc.

Sunday is your reward day. So enjoy it.

***

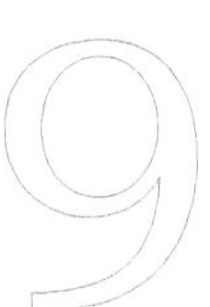

# SUPPLEMENTS / NUTRITION

**P**rotein shakes, weight loss pills, green tea, appetite blockers, carb blocker, fat burners, CLA and many more products....  Sports Nutrition is a huge industry.

They use the most scientific words to describe the high tech weapons that should help you to fight your fat.

And every few months a new wonder product hits the shelves.

They promise short term results and a convenient way to achieve your goals.

But is it the right way? Here is my opinion.

I have tested a lot over the last two decades for gaining muscles, strength and losing fat. I have wasted a lot of money. And I talked a lot to professional athletes and bodybuilders.

99% of the products are bogus. They might not harm you, but they do not really help at all. In the long run they might even have dangerous consequences.

What they do is that, they help to fill the pockets of the Sports Nutrition companies.

So you can go for proteins like Whey protein and diet protein bars if you can afford it.

You can also go for multivitamin tabs. No problem at

all. I take Omega Fish Oil Tabs myself.

Everything else you can try, but I can guarantee you that it will not give you a real deal for your money.

This book is about being healthy and it is not about hardcore ways to get hardcore results like professional bodybuilders do.

And even though hardcore bodybuilders might be impressive, believe me: they are living really unhealthy. If it is done incorrectly it could even kill you. So let's leave this to the freaks.

You can only lose fat, if you burn more energy that you eat.

Now we have optimized your eating habits and your food choice.

This means that you will eat more often, fewer calories, better and healthier food and maybe have a higher water intake. But we have only adjusted one of the variables.

The other variable is the energy that your body burns over the day. If you have an office job then you will probably be sitting for many hours each day.

This means that you will not burn much energy automatically, which in turn means that you have to do some exercise to get your body to burn fat.

***

# 10

# THE TRAINING

Yes, this is not a diet only concept. We will also do some exercise to get you into shape.

It is a 6 day on, 1 day off scheme. So we train 6 days and day number 7 is free. No sports, nada...

The training is split into 3 days of cardiovascular

training and 3 days of weightlifting and fitness training.

On Mondays, Wednesdays and Fridays you will do your weightlifting work outs.

On Tuesday, Thursdays and Saturdays you will do your cardio days.

And Sunday again is your rest day.

The following pages will give you some general information about the training and will show you a training week which you can use as an example.

Generally it is a good idea to warm up your body first. So start light with cardio or weights for a few minutes and sets. After the training take a couple of minutes to cool down. You can do this easily by doing a few stretching exercises on a mat.

If your home or gym provides a sauna or a steam bath, you should use this once or twice a week. And remember to drink enough water (water, nothing else), especially directly after your work out.

The start might be hard at first, but after a few weeks your training should be an integral part of your live just as brushing your teeth in the morning is.

Due to the fact that you should do your training directly after you get out of bed it might be harder in wintertime when it is still dark outside.

But in the summer it is just great. You will feel much better and revitalized when you go to work.

***

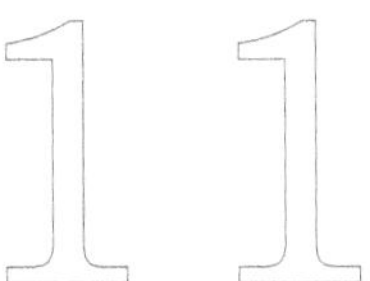

# YOUR CARDIOVASCLUAR TRAINING

**H**ere is the trick: You are going to burn the fat when your body is in a situation that he needs to burn it. And this in the morning.

The explanation is easy:

You have your last low carb meal at 9.00pm. So in

the night while you are asleep, you body will burn all carbohydrates that are available to maintain body temperature, recover cells and to move you in your sleep.

In the morning your body is waiting for its breakfast as the carb resources are most likely almost empty.

Now you give it only a glass of water and some fat burning supplements, that will boost your metabolism to burn fat and then you enter the treadmill, start your training bike or start your morning run.

So instead of filling up the empty storages, you will burn even more energy. To boost your start you can also drink a coffee (no sugar!) first, but do not forget to drink your glass of water.

It is important that you do your exercise in a pulse range of about 140 beats per minute and for at least 20-30 min. Do warm up some minutes (important) and then bring your pulse to a constant 140bpm.

After 30 min (40 min if you like) you are done and

then you can go for a shower and next thing is breakfast.

That is basically your cardio work out. Of course you can add more cardio works outs if you want. But the ones in the morning are the most important ones.

And during the day you can follow some easy and effective tricks to burn more calories.

- Take the stairs instead the escalator or elevator.

- If you have an office job, take some time during the day to go outside and to stretch a bit. Instead of joining the smokers club you should take a stroll around the block.

- If you have a dog, walk it one hour per day. If you do not have one you could maybe ask the neighbor if you can walk their dog. It is always more interesting to walk with a purpose instead of walking alone.

- Think about other ways to increase the amount of kilometers that you walk. Try to walk at least 8000 steps (7 km) a day; on weekends try to walk more than this. Explore the forest, mountain or beach trials in your area.

- Get yourself an electronic step counter, to track your daily steps and your progress. If you have a Nokia Smartphone like a Nokia N95 it supplies free software called Step Counter that I can recommend.

You can even attach it to your cell phone GPS and then you also know where you are walking. You should know this anyhow ;-), but at least then you cannot get lost.

***

# YOUR WEIGHTLIFTING WORKOUT

The cardiovascular training helps to burn fat, but you need to train your muscles from different angles. And you need to form and shape your muscles. For every pound of muscle you add, your body will burn 50 more calories per day!  Weightlifting is the perfect counterpart to your cardio workout.

The way to do this is to do moderate weight training.

Again, this book is not about turning you into a world class bodybuilder or a super strong weightlifter.
It will only show you how you can achieve the best for your life.

It would be good, if you are a member in a gym. If not, you need to have a home-gym and the equipment. This is most likely an expensive investment. A gym membership has simply more advantages.

What you can do is get yourself a treadmill or a stationary bike and do your cardio days at home. Then you only need to go to the gym for your weightlifting days. That might save you some time, if a gym is not nearby.

If you arrive at the gym, then start to train immediately. Do not fool yourself and chat to people or stay at the juice bar all the time.

Avoid talking a lot to people (only when you need help). Once your training is done you can socialize.

# YOUR WEIGHTLIFTING WORKOUT

With this training program you do not need to spend long hours in the gym. The entire training program per day should be done within 30-40 minutes.
So your weight training day will not take longer than your cardio training day.

You should split the body groups into 3 training days, in other words: You train your whole body once a week.

The training plan is only an example. You will find huge amounts of websites that supply you with training plans. Stick to this basic training for at least four weeks.

You can then start to add other exercises to the training. This will ensure that your training does not become boring.

As there are more than 700 exercises in weightlifting you should visit this website for some ideas:
http://www.exrx.net/Lists/Directory.html

You see that we use sets and reps (repetitions). This

means that your should do a certain exercise for example 2 times (sets) and each time you do the movements for example 12 times (reps).

We start the week with leg training. There is a simple reason for this.

Usually the gyms are fully packed on Monday and for some reason, everybody starts with chest training on Mondays.

So you will have to cue in for certain exercises. Due to the fact that we do not want to lose time, we therefore start with the leg training.

Here is your training plan.

**Monday – weight training - quadriceps, hamstrings and calves**

Quadriceps:
- Leg Extensions 2 Sets x 12 Reps
- Leg Presses 1 x 12, 1 x 10, 1 x 8, 1 x 6, 1 x 12 Reps

Increase the weight on each set and lower it for the

last set.

Hamstrings:

* Lying Leg Curls 4 x 12 Reps

Calves:

* Seated Calf Raises  4 x 15 Reps
* or Standing Heel Raises 4 x 15 Reps

Try increasing your weight on each set, but keep control over the weight all the time and focus on the correct technique.

Abs:

* Floor Crunches  4 x 20 Reps

Done. This should not take longer than 30 to 40 minutes. Push yourself as hard as possible, but always focus on the correct technique.

## Tuesday - cardiovascular training

On Tuesdays you do your cardiovascular training for example 20 min on the stationary bike and 10 min on the treadmill.

Remember that you pulse after the warm up should stay at around 140 beats per minute.

## Wednesday – weight training - chest, shoulder and triceps

This time we train the chest, shoulder and triceps.

Chest:

- Barbell Bench Press 1 x 12, 1 x 10, 1 x 8, 1 x 6, 1 x 12 Reps (Increase the weight on each set and lower it for the last set.)
- Dumbbell Flyes 4 x 10 Reps

Shoulders:

- Seated Dumbbell Press  1 x 12, 1 x 10, 1 x 8, 1 x 12 Reps
- Upright Barbell Rows 4 x 10 Reps

Triceps:

- Bench Dips 4 x 10 Reps
- Triceps Pushdowns 1 x 10, 1 x 8, 1 x 6 Reps, 1 x 12 Reps (Increase the weight on each set and lower it for the last set.)

Abs:

- Floor Crunches  4 x 20 Reps

## Thursday - cardiovascular training

On Thursday you do your cardiovascular training for example 20 min on the stepper and 10 min on the treadmill. Remember that you pulse after the warm up should stay at around 140 beats per minute.

## Friday – weight training – back and biceps

Friday is the last weight training day for the week. This time we hit your back and biceps.

Back:

- Wide-Grip Lat Pulldown 1 x 12, 1 x 10, 1 x 8, 1 x 6, 1 x 12 Reps (Increase the weight on each set and lower it for the last set.)
- Seated Cable Rows 4 x 10 Reps

Biceps:

- Alternate Dumbbell Curls 4 x 12

- Hammer Curls 2 x 10

Abs:

- Floor Crunches  4 x 20 Reps

Done.

## Saturday - cardiovascular training

On Saturdays you do your cardiovascular training for example 20 min on the treadmill and 10 min on the stationary bike. Remember that you pulse after the warm up should stay at around 140 beats per minute.

## Sunday – no training

Have a rest and enjoy your "all you can eat" day. And on Monday start again with the training!!!

***

13

# YOUR WORKOUT LOG

It is a good idea to write your workouts into a training log. This will help you to remember what exercise you did at your last training and how much weight you have used.

Below you will find a very basic workout log. You can easily create something like this in Excel or just got to Google and search for "workout log xls". You will get plenty of files that you can use.

A training log is also fun because you to look back on your old logs and see what you used to do way back when!

At this website you can create your personal training log even online:
http://www.bodybuilding.com/fun/printworklog.htm

Example of a workout log:

| EXERCISES | SETS | REPS | WT |
| --- | --- | --- | --- |
|  |  |  |  |

# 14

# USEFUL BOOKS AND LINKS

The Internet is full of information about diets, training and work out plans. But you actually do not need much of this.

Have a look at these 3 websites and which will give you more information than you ever will need to reach your goal.

http://bodyforlife.com/ - Body for life - Basically the foundation of my training plan but note that you do not need to train every body part twice a week and you do not spend all your money on the products of this sports nutrition supplier.

There are also some books available:

- Body for Life: 12 Weeks to Mental and Physical Strength, Bill Phillips, ISBN-13: 978-0060193393

- Eating For Life, Bill Phillips, ISBN-13: 978-0972018418

- Body-for-LIFE for Women: A Woman's Plan for Physical and Mental Transformation, Dr. Pamela Peeke, ISBN-13: 978-1605298283

- The Men's Health Big Book of Exercises: Four Weeks to a Leaner, Stronger, More Muscular YOU!, Adam Campbell, ISBN-13: 978-1605295503

- The Greatness Guide: 101 Lessons for Making What's Good at Work and in Life Even Better, Robin Sharma, ISBN-13: 978-0061238574

- The Greatness Guide, Book 2: 101 Lessons for Success and Happiness, Robin Sharma, ISBN-13: 978-1554684038

And one book that explains every possible aspect of bodybuilding:

- The New Encyclopedia of Modern Bodybuilding: The Bible of Bodybuilding, Fully Updated and Revised by Arnold Schwarzenegger and Bill Dobbins, ISBN-13: 978-0684857213

These websites give you some very good information on healthy eating and training:

Just Enough for You: About Food Portions
http://win.niddk.nih.gov/publications/just_enough.htm

Nutrition for Everyone
http://www.cdc.gov/nutrition/everyone/index.html

How to Understand & Use the Nutrition Facts Label, http://www.fda.gov/Food/LabelingNutrition/Consu merInformation/ucm078889.htm

Healthy Eating for Weight Loss http://women.webmd.com/guide/nutrition-101-how-to-eat-healthy

Men's Health - Men's Guide to Fitness, Health, Weight Loss, Nutrition. Lots of stuff to read and you learn a lot about living a healthy lifestyle. http://www.menshealth.com/men/ -

Project Weight Loss - Weight loss community featuring a BMI calculator, calorie counter, menu planner, workout planner, and more! http://www.projectweightloss.com

Jillian Michael's weight loss program takes into account three factors - self, science, and sweat. http://www.jillianmichaels.com/

BodyDæmon offers a free Online Fitness Journal that will change the way you think about, share and record your health. http://www.bodydaemon.com/

***

15

# CONCLUSION

This book is intended as a quick start for you to lose fat, gain muscles and start a healthier lifestyle.

It only covers the basics. There is definitely more information available in other books and the Internet but this book is more than enough information to start right away.

If you want to learn about the complicated processes that happen in your body or you want the full overview of all possible exercises then you will need books with hundreds of pages.

You can read these books while you have already started with my program and it is a good idea to do this while doing your cardio training while you are already on the way.

Let me know, how the program works for you and if you have achieved your goal.

Stay focused and be disciplined. The first few weeks will be the hardest part. Once you have managed this, it will be much easier. And believe me. Everyone can do this!!

Please feel free to visit the online reader's forum of this book and discuss your questions about food, diet and training with other readers and me, the author.

Let this book grow with your experience, tips and ideas.

CONCLUSION

Visit my blog for my daily updates on diet and training at http://its-a-guys-world.com/category/health/

You can post your questions on the online forum of the book and discuss topics with other readers at: http://its-a-guys-world.com/community/

Also please feel free to follow and contact me at:

Email: blog@its-a-guys-world.com
RSS News Feed: http://its-a-guys-world.com/feed/
Twitter: http://www.twitter.com/guznuname
MySpace: http://www.myspace.com/claus-lauter
Facebook: http://www.facebook.com/claus.lauter
XING: http://www.xing.com/profile/Claus_Lauter
Linkedin: http://za.linkedin.com/in/southafrica

# 16

# SHARING THIS DOCUMENT

There was a lot of work that went into putting this document together. That means that this information has value, and your friends, neighbors, and co-workers may want to share it.

The information in this document is copyrighted. I would ask that you do not share this information with others. You purchased this book, and you have a right to use.

Another person who has not purchased this book does not have that right. It is in the sales of this valuable information that makes the continued publishing of this book possible. If enough people disregard that simple economic fact then the book will no longer be viable or available.

If your friends think this information is valuable enough to ask you for it then they should think it is valuable enough to purchase it themselves. After all, the price is low enough that just about anyone should be able to afford it.

It should go without saying that you cannot post this document or the information it contains on any electronic bulletin board, Web site, FTP site, newsgroup, or ... well, you get the idea.

The only source from which this document should be available is the website of the author. If you want an original copy, visit the website at the following address: http://www.its-a-guys-world.com

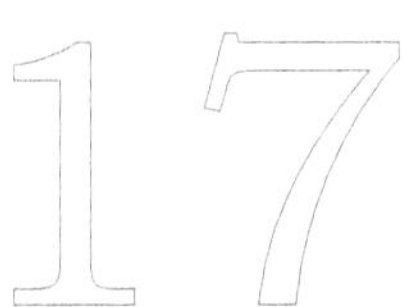

# LEGAL NOTICE

Limit of Liability and Disclaimer of Warranty: The author has used his best efforts in preparing this book, and the information provided herein is provided "as is".

The author makes no representation or warranties with respect to the accuracy or completeness of the contents of this book and specifically disclaims any

# LEGAL NOTICE

implied warranties of merchantability or fitness for any particular purpose and shall in no event be liable for any loss of profit or any other commercial damage, including but not limited to special, incidental, consequential, or other damages.

Trademarks: This book identifies product names and services known to be trademarks, registered trademarks, or service marks of their respective holders.

They are used throughout this book in an editorial fashion only. In addition, terms suspected of being trademarks, registered trademarks, or service marks have been appropriately capitalized, although the author cannot attest to the accuracy of this information.

The use of a term in this book should not be regarded as affecting the validity of any trademark, registered trademark, or service mark.

The author is not associated with any product or vendor mentioned in this book.

Some links within this book may lead to websites, including those operated and maintained by third parties.

The author includes these links solely as a convenience to you, and the presence of such a link does not imply a responsibility for the linked site or an endorsement of the linked site, its operator, or its contents (exceptions may apply).

***

18

# DISCLAIMER

The content of this book describes depicts ways to lose fat and shape your body.

The diet and training scheme worked as well for the author as for numerous other people who were introduced to this plan trough the writer.

Although there is no guarantee that this will also

work for you, there is a very high chance that it will.

The author is not a medical doctor or physiologist so all advise given in this book are simply approved by more than 20 years of fitness training experience by the writer.

You should always consult your doctor for a general check-up and get advise if you are allowed to start a cardiovascular and weightlifting program.

You should also consult your doctor before making drastic changes to your diet and your lifestyle, especially if you take medication of any kind.

Keep in mind that nutritional needs vary from person to person, depending on age, sex health status and total diet.

Finally you should also consult a private trainer or a trainer in a gym to let him show you the correct technique of exercises and how to operate machines like treadmills. If you injure yourself due to a lack of technique, it will be your fault and your fault only.

# DISCLAIMER

Your reliance upon information and content obtained by you at or through this publication is solely at your own risk.

The author assumes no liability or responsibility for damage or injury to you, other persons, or property arising from any use of any product, information, idea, or instruction contained in the content or services provided to you through this book.

The author has no financial interest in and receives no compensation from manufacturers of products or websites mentioned in this book.

***

# 18

# ABOUT THE AUTHOR

The author is a Natural Bodybuilder and has started his sports 1987 at the age of 19.

He has a certificate as Fitness Trainer and has completed an apprenticeship as a chef (cook).

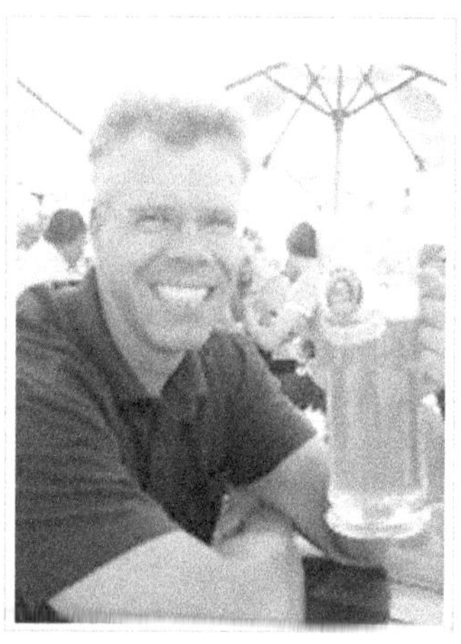

He was born and raised in Germany and after extensive traveling he now lives and works in Cape Town, South Africa.

He is the Marketing Director for a company called Intergate Immigration and helps people and companies with their move to South Africa.

He has never taken any steroids or other anabolic substances, as it was never his intention to compete on stage with other bodybuilders.

He has trained in gyms all over the world and had the chance to meet some of the leading fitness and bodybuilding professionals.

His is 183cm tall and his max. weight was 103 kg. Today his weight is between 83-87kg with 12-14% body fat. He still enjoys a glass of beer (picture) or wine and his favorite is Italian and Asian food.

Now at an age above 40 and with more than 20 years experience in natural bodybuilding and fitness training, he likes to share his experience with others.

# INDEX

# INDEX